Soft Media Publishing Presents

How To Get a Miracle

"Discover The Secret Law In Quantum Physics Cracked The Miracle Code"!

Whether you need a healing in your body or a boost in your finances the revelations in this book will change your life forever.

The author takes you step by step through scientifically documented principles and newly discovered laws that open up unlimited possibilities for your future.

Discover for yourself how secret but proven age old wisdom combined with scientific research has unlocked the hidden mysteries of the universe!

Table of Contents

"An uplifting and empowering book. This very well written book is perfect for anyone looking to take control of their future rather than just being a participant in it!" ~Christian Marshall

"This is a very beneficial read. This book will help you attain and live life with less stress. Change to a life with more positive energy, starting right now, with small actionable steps. I have made it a daily practice and refer to the book regularly... creating positive emotions. I am already noticing the health benefits!" ~S.Y. Ward, R.N."

"Hello Grey, Wow! Your writing is very inspiring... In school, I had a teacher who discouraged me by saying that miracles do not exist. She actually gave a lecture on this theory. I am glad that your book disproved her." ~Morissa Schwartz: senior at The Middlesex Academy for Allied Health and Biomedical Science

Chapter 1

The Miracles of Yesterday are the Science of Today

Have you been searching for the answers to life's greatest questions? Maybe you've been looking for answers in the books you've read or the movies you've seen.

Possibly you've been looking at the teachings of various religions and have pieces of the puzzle, but you're still unable to see the whole picture.

The fact that you are here now reading this... is no accident!

In this book, you'll discover the secret to unlocking the doors of health, wealth and abundance in every area of your life.

Miracles are real and they are available to anyone who learns and applies the revelations set forth in this book.

The world as you know it, is about to change before your very eyes forever, if you have an open mind and if you are a seeker of truth.

Scientific advancements are unraveling the mysteries of the universe as never before seen in the history of mankind.

Inside the pages of this book, exists an incredible life changing power, that is available to all who hold the key and aren't afraid to use it!

This incredible power literally shapes and forms the very fabric of our universe and even transcends time and space.

You will discover that your perceptions, and the way you interpret reality...within the deepest core of your being...is the very matrix from which flows all health, wealth and abundance.

You'll discover scientifically, that your physical body and everything that surrounds you, is not solid, but consists of moving vibrating energy fields.

These energy fields can be influenced positively or negatively by this age old wisdom, to dramatically alter the course of your life.

These energy fields are subject to specific laws and hidden principles that when understood and applied have the power to transform your life from the average into the miraculous.

Chapter 2

Miracles Are Created

Yes, you read that right...miracles are created! Whether you need a miracle in your body or in your finances, the principles are the same.

Have you ever wondered why some people get miracles while others don't?

Would you like to know the secret of how some amass great wealth, while others barely survive? How is it that if you give two people the exact same business opportunity, one becomes wildly successful while the other goes broke?

Even when they follow the same business plan!

I'm going to show you newly discovered scientifically proven truths that take the miraculous out of the realm of the supernatural, and place it squarely within your grasp.

What you do with these incredible amazing truths is up to you.

I'll show you in easy to follow segments, how miracles can be created by anyone, if they have a strong desire to learn, understand and apply this ancient wisdom.

You'll see firsthand how Quantum Physics has cracked the miracle code and made accessing a miracle, something that anyone can understand!

Let's get started by taking a look at a documented healing miracle.

In the movie The Secret, Cathy Goodman, a young lady who had a doctor verified case of breast cancer, was completely healed.

She didn't take chemotherapy or radiation, and over a period of three months, her cancer disappeared and her Doctors gave her a clean bill of health!

She states that she believed in her heart that she was already healed.

She would spend the day in a posture of gratefulness and declare out loud..."Thank you for my healing"...over and over again.

She visualized herself as if cancer was never in her body. She watched funny movies and laughed all the time.

She realized she couldn't afford to have any stress in her life, so she eliminated anything that she considered stressful, that would cause her to feel negative emotions such as fear or anger.

As you go through this book, you'll see scientifically what happened in Cathy's life that created her miracle,

You'll discover how to use the same scientifically proven principles, to generate a miracle for health or finances, in your life when you need one.

After years of investigation into miracles, healings, and the study of Quantum Physics, I've discovered why some get miracles while others don't.

As you begin to understand the truths and principles that are revealed in this book, you'll have a step by step blueprint into the realm of the miraculous.
Keep an open mind, and don't let your old beliefs stop you from receiving these scientifically proven principles.

If you can do that, you'll be awed and amazed with the results, and you'll enter into a whole new realm of possibilities for your life!

Ok let's get started.

If you wanted to build a house the first thing you would do is to begin to imagine what your house would look like.

You would begin to visualize in your minds eye, all the features you want in your new house.

Then you would hire an architect to help you put down on paper the layout and all the details like size, materials etc. or you would find a similar plan that someone else visualized and created from their imagination.

Then you would hire a contractor, purchase materials and the house would be built according to your specifications.

This chain of events is the same process, whether you are building a house, making furniture, manufacturing a car or concocting the latest pharmaceutical to sell to the masses.

Everything we create starts as an idea that we visualize or imagine in our mind. Every idea begins in the unseen invisible realm of our thoughts and imaginations.

In other words you can't touch taste or smell an idea.

Ideas are invisible!

We all know ideas are real even if we can't see them because we all have them.

The first step in learning to live in the miraculous is to understand the world, the universe literally everything we see was made the same way.

Just as a building requires a design and a builder, the world, the universe and everything in them, also demands a Creator.

Dave Hunt, speaker, radio commentator and author, makes an excellent argument regarding creationism.

He states there had to be someone, not something (things wear out... 2nd law of thermo dynamics) without beginning or end.

This someone had to have the power, the wisdom and the infinite intelligence to engineer, integrate and harmonize every part of the creation... from the organization of the atom, to the creation of the universe.

Hunt goes on to say, we all begin as a single cell the size of a period like the one at the end of this sentence.

He explains that this cell goes on to build a complete body with over 100 trillion cells in it, composed of thousands of different kinds of cells.

He poses the question, "How does that one little cell know how to build a body with over 100 trillion cells in it?

Each one of those cells is so complex nano chemical machinery, that even today, in this scientifically advanced age we live in, understanding & duplicating something as simple as the cell, is far beyond mankind's abilities

Let's go deeper.

DNA is another extremely compelling proof that there has to be a Creator.

Did you know that DNA is the densest storage mechanism in the universe?

The amount of information contained in a pinhead volume of DNA, would fill a stack of books 500 times higher than from here to the moon!

Ken Ham President of Answers in Genesis explains that the DNA in our genes are like books of information, that's read by a language system.

Ham goes on to say, "scientists know today that language as a code only comes from intelligence.

No one has ever seen matter by itself give rise to a code. Nobody has ever seen matter by itself give rise to information."

This means that since language as a code comes from intelligence, and our DNA are like books of information, that's read by a language system, means we were created by an Intelligence!

This is scientific proof that we were created by intelligence, and this fact is paramount to understanding how miracles work.

Chapter 3

What is a Miracle?

In order for us to be able to live in the miraculous, we first need to understand what a miracle is.

Dictionary.com defines a miracle as: An effect or extraordinary event in the physical world that surpasses all known human or natural powers, and is ascribed to a supernatural cause.

According to that definition... a miracle is something that we can never understand or depend on...

The term miracle is really just a word we use to describe something we don't understand. `

In this book I will prove to you that a miracle is simply the ability to understand laws that our Creator put in place to hold creation together.

Also I would like to point out, you don't need to understand these laws to make them work for us, but I do feel the more we understand how these laws work, the easier it will be to get them.

There was a time that the thought of someone flying through the air would have been considered a miracle.

Today we know that man flying through the air isn't a miracle, but simply the harnessing and application of the laws of Newtonian Physics!

Newtonian Physics is the study of how the physical things that we can see all around us work.

When Newton, the father of physics, was sitting under the apple tree he noticed the law of gravity while he watched an apple fall to the ground.

Here is the exact story as related from Newton to his friend Stukeley:
"After dinner, the weather being warm, we went into the garden and drank tea, under the shade of some apple trees... he told me, he was just in the same situation, as when formerly, the notion of gravitation came into his mind.

It was occasioned by the fall of an apple, as he sat in contemplative mood.

Why should that apple always descend perpendicularly to the ground, thought he to himself..."

Newtonian Physics is simply the understanding and application of laws such as the law of gravity.

We call these laws because they work every time!

As mankind began to understand the laws of Newtonian Physics, flying was no longer in the realm of the miraculous, but simply the understanding and application of scientifically proven laws.

Does this mean that our Creator had nothing to do with this miracle?

Absolutely not... He put ALL laws into existence, when He created the world and the universe.

Our Creator had everything to do with it.

Everything in creation operates under specifically designed laws... EVERYTHING!

I will prove scientifically to you that a miracle is simply the ability to operate within laws that have been with us since the dawn of creation.

In this book I'm going to prove to you, that a miracle is not something we can't understand and just happens out of nowhere.

I'm even going to show you how you can use these newly discovered laws, to access the realm of the miraculous on a daily basis.

In fact I'm going to go so far as to say that once you learn to master these mysterious laws... nothing will be impossible for you!

Chapter 4

Without Laws Creation Couldn't Exist

Creation exists and operates under specific laws that were implemented by our Creator.

Without laws nothing in this world would be able to function consistently in a predictable manner.

Without the absolute consistency of laws... we wouldn't be able to leverage these laws to our advantage and achieve the technological advances we enjoy today.

Without laws, the world would literally fall apart...nothing could survive!

Let's take a look at the definition of a law, as in a scientific setting.

Merriam-Webster defines a law as: a rule of construction or procedure.

When our Creator made creation He obviously used laws as a rule of construction.

For example, in order for us to be able to stay on this earth and not float off into space He used the law of gravity, as a rule of construction.

Many of our Creators laws have been hidden from our eyes in a scientific sense, until the last hundred years or so.

We are really just beginning to uncover and understand, some of these laws.

The laws of creation are so exact, that as we understand and work with them, we are able to fly planes through the air, track people's location using GPS, and communicate instantly around the world with anyone.

Most of the laws we understand, operate through Newtonian Physics, the physical realm of earth and universe that we can see, feel and hear with our physical senses.

There are also laws that operate through Quantum Physics, the unseen realm of the microscopic.

Quantum Physics is simply the study of the sub atomic world, as seen through the eyes of an electron microscope.

Quantum Physics is the study of the unseen realm.

Remember in the previous chapter we proved that ideas begin in the unseen realm of our imagination?

We are just beginning to discover and understand how some of the laws in the quantum realm work.

The study of Quantum Physics is revealing to us, what the fabric of the universe, the world and literally the entire Creation consists of.

Quantum Physics is answering questions mankind has had since the dawn of creation.

What we are also discovering is that the laws of Newtonian Physics operate much differently than the laws of Quantum Physics.

Chapter 5

Quantum Physics the Window into the Unseen Realm

In order to understand the mechanics of a miracle, it is crucial to have a basic understanding of Quantum Physics.

Don't worry, this isn't as complicated as it sounds, and I promise I won't bore you.

Quantum Physics is simply the scientific study of the Creation at the sub atomic level.

In other words, Quantum Physics is the study of the unseen realm... or as I mentioned above...the study of the creation, as seen through the eyes of a very powerful electron microscope.

This amazing sub atomic world, is revealing to anyone who will listen, secrets that transcend time and space.

This knowledge helps us understand the mechanics of a miracle and how miracles are created.

Quantum Physics has proven that the universe, the world and everything we can see touch and feel, is not solid but consists entirely of energy fields!

Here is a quote from the father of Quantum Physics, Max Plank, a theoretical physicist who originated quantum theory, which won him the Nobel Prize in Physics in 1918.

Quote: **"As a man who has devoted his whole life to the most clear headed science, to the study of matter, I can tell you as a result of my research about atoms this much:**

There is no matter as such.

All matter originates and exists only by virtue of a force which brings the particle of an atom to vibration and holds this most minute solar system of the atom together.

We must assume behind this force the existence of a conscious and intelligent mind.

This mind is the matrix of all matter." end quote

Did you get that?

Everything is energy and it is controlled by a conscious and intelligent Mind!

The chair you sit in, the car you drive, the pets in your house and even your physical body, is not made up of of anything solid.

Everything consists of energy field's, that are compacted and configured together in such a way, that we can see and interact with them.

Why is this important?

Because, it has been proven that when a scientist does an experiment at the quantum level, what he or she BELIEVES about the results of that experiment, will influence the energy fields at the quantum level, changing the outcome of that experiment!

Did you catch that?

The **BELIEF** of any person conducting an experiment at the quantum level **will influence the outcome of the experiment.**

Here is a quote from Som.org

"At the level of the quark, scientists have experienced confusing results in the data that they have received from their experiments in regard to their direction and velocity of movement...

Quarks have exhibited movement based upon the thoughts and expectations of the scientists involved in the respective experiments" end quote

Quantum Physics is showing us that anything we truly BELIEVE at the core of our being... in our hearts, has the power to change or alter the energy fields inside us... and the energy fields in the world around us!

Quantum Physics has proven that our organs, tissues, bones, literally our entire being... is simply configured energy fields.

So what you and I believe about ourselves and the world around us, changes the energy fields in our bodies and the world around us, for good or bad

If we have negative beliefs about ourselves and the world around us... our physical bodies and the world around us will change to conform to those beliefs.

I'm going to prove to you that BELIEF is the main law or rule of construction that our Creator put in place for everything to run smoothly in His creation.

The study of Quantum Physics is revealing to us different kinds of laws than the ones we are used to operating under.

This is earth shattering news, because according to Quantum Physics, everything that happens at the quantum level manifests itself in this physical world of sight sound and touch.

Chapter 6

Believe It or Not

Your health, your prosperity, your relationships... everything you are, or ever hope to be is all controlled and held together by your belief system!

Everyone has a belief system of one kind or another.

The important thing to understand here is... whatever belief system that has formed in you, will ultimately dictate the quality of life you live, according to Quantum Physics.

And I don't mean believing in your head... I mean believing in your heart... the very core of your being.

There's a huge difference.

We all believe one thing or another.

It's critical that we develop a belief system that will generate a full healthy abundant life.

If we don't become active participants in developing our belief system, we'll be like a ship at sea without a rudder to steer us.

We need to eliminate all the harmful beliefs in us that are poisoning our lives and the lives of those we love.

We MUST focus on replacing those old harmful toxic beliefs with life giving, healthy positive beliefs.

What I'm saying here is if we want prosperity and health we shouldn't choose a belief system that encourages poverty and sickness.

One of the reasons I chose the teachings of the Bible was because our Creator, at the very beginning of the Bible, paints a solid picture of the kind of life He wants for His Creation.

He placed man in an amazing paradise He called the Garden of Eden and surrounded Adam and Eve with eternal life, perfect health and abundance.

There was no sickness or disease... there was no poverty... there was no lack or death... there was no sorrow!

So my conclusion has to be, according to the Bible, that the ultimate purpose our Creator had in mind for His creation was exactly that, eternal life, perfect health and abundance.

If my life is filled with sickness, disease and poverty, I need to align myself and my belief system... with the Creator of life, health and abundance.

The teachings of the Bible have everything in a belief system that is necessary to succeed in all areas of life.

In fact the Bible is exploding with the laws of Quantum Physics!

These laws are much different than the laws we are familiar with in Newtonian Physics, such as the law of gravity.

The Bible teaches us how to reap the benefits that the laws of Quantum Physics offer us, without the need to understand the science behind Quantum Physics.

But we are so very privileged at this time in history, to also have the science of Quantum Physics available, to verify Gods Word.

The laws of Quantum Physics are at work everywhere in the Bible and confirm the teachings of the Bible at every turn!

You may ask yourself why then are so many Christians sick and broke?

Speaking from personal experience, I'm going to go out on a limb here and say it's because of unbelief (belief in something else) or not having knowledge of what is available to us.

Let me explain.

The Bible says in Philippians 4:19 And my God shall supply all your need according to His riches in glory by Christ Jesus.

If I say that I believe that to be true, and suddenly a bill comes due and the money isn't in my account to pay that bill.

I can and have... gone into panic mode, which shows me that I don't believe God in this area.

As a matter of fact, if I'm being truthful to myself, my true heart core belief is that He won't meet my need!

Unbelief is simply the belief in something else.

We all have the ability to give mental assent to an idea in our conscious mind, without truly believing that idea in such a way that it changes our lives at the very heart or core of our being.

In fact we can even convince ourselves that we believe something when we really don't.

Quantum laws are influenced by our thoughts, emotions and beliefs, which will ultimately manifest their results in this physical world and affect our lives for positive or negative.

As we know, you can't see your thoughts or beliefs, but because we all have them, we know they are real.

Since the quantum world is the unseen realm, and our thoughts and beliefs, (though invisible) have been proven to influence the unseen realm, we can say that our thoughts and beliefs operate at the quantum level.

So...what you and I believe in our hearts about anything, whether we like it or not, those beliefs will trigger laws at the quantum level for good or for bad in our lives.

Have you ever noticed that if you are afraid of something it tends to come to pass in your life?

For instance if you have a feeling that something you are doing will fail... it usually does. Conversely when you know deep down inside you that you will succeed, you do!

Chapter 7

Energy Flows Where Attention Goes

Are you getting it?

What you think and believe about yourself, your abilities and even your health or your finances have been scientifically proven to alter you and the things around you!

You and I are the result of what we truly believe about ourselves down deep in the inner core of our being.

Everyone operates their entire lives through a belief system of one kind or another.

So whether you are an Atheist, Buddhist, Islamic, Hindu, Christian or whatever religion you believe in, how you are taught, and how you interpret and take to heart the teachings of your religion, according to Quantum Physics, will ultimately alter your life, health and even your physical surroundings.

It's important to understand that the laws or rules of construction our Creator used, when He designed creation, allow for higher laws to override lower laws.

Let me give you an example.

If you threw a person off the Empire State Building the law of gravity doesn't care if they're a good person or a bad person, they will hit the ground and die.

But the law of gravity can be overridden by a higher law, the law of lift.

So if you take that same person and put him on a plane, (whether he is a good person or bad) he will be able to fly over any building and gravity won't be able to stop him.

Let's look at a higher law overriding a lower law at the quantum level, in the Bible.

Romans 8:2 for the law of the Spirit of life in Christ Jesus has made me free from the law of sin and death.

So the Bible is saying there is a law of the Spirit of life in Christ Jesus, and a law of sin and death, and that the law of the Spirit of life in Christ Jesus is a higher law that overrides the law of sin and death.

The law of the Spirit of life in Christ Jesus and the law of sin and death are two separate laws, and one law overrides the other, just as the law of lift overrides the law of gravity.

The law of life and the law of sin and death are unseen laws that manifest themselves in Newtonian Physics (the world we see feel and touch) but these laws are rooted in the quantum realm (the unseen microscopic world where everything is energy.)

All of the laws in the Bible have their roots exclusively in the quantum (unseen) realm.

These quantum laws are laws that science isn't used to seeing, understanding or explaining, but scientists are beginning to understand some of them.

As in the above example of throwing someone off the Empire State building, whether we recognize the law of gravity or not, we will fall to the ground every time, proving the law.

So even if we don't understand or even recognize all the laws in the quantum unseen realm, our Creator has put in place, these quantum laws are still laws, and they work for us or against us, whether we understand them or not.

Do these laws work for everyone even if they don't believe in God?

A law is a law and always does what a law was created to do.

Many people have used Gods laws for personal gain, and to fulfill selfish desires and ambitions.

They have even had the ability to accomplish what we might call supernatural events, without ever accepting God for who He is.

Let me give you an example from the Bible

Exodus 7:10 And Aaron cast down his rod before Pharaoh and before his servants, and it became a serpent.

11 But Pharaoh also called the wise men and the sorcerers; so the magicians of Egypt, they also did in like manner with their enchantments.

12 For every man threw down his rod, and they became serpents. But Aaron's rod swallowed up their rods. (Proving who was stronger)

It's important here to remember that God knew man would learn to manipulate His laws, and so He created higher laws to override lower laws.

He made it so that mankind can only go so far manipulating laws for selfish gain or to even harm others.

The only way anyone can experience full abundant life here in this life and eternal life in the life to come, is through operating in the higher law of the Spirit of life in Christ Jesus thereby overriding the law of sin and death.

There is only one way to operate in this higher law of the Spirit of life in Christ Jesus and that's by sincerely asking Jesus to be our Lord and Savior, as our deepest hearts cry!

Romans 10:9 that if you confess with your mouth the Lord Jesus and believe in your heart that God has raised Him from the dead, you will be saved.

You just can't fake a decision like that.

Chapter 8

The Law of Belief

Belief is the core quantum law upon which all other laws of creation (rules of construction) hinge.

In the Garden of Eden before the fall, everything worked in perfect harmony. Nothing was out of sync and would have continued perfectly forever because no laws had been broken.

Adam and Eve had no understanding of good and evil and the condemnation guilt and shame that came along with this knowledge.

They were blissfully ignorant regarding right and wrong and had perfect fellowship with our Creator because they believed everything He told them.

They knew God had said in Genesis 2:17…"but of the tree of the knowledge of good and evil you shall not eat, for in the day that you eat of it you shall surely die."

That was fine with them because they believed God and hadn't even considered that God would say something that wasn't true, but they always had a choice because God doesn't want robots.

He gave Adam and Eve the ability to choose for themselves what they wanted to believe.

So when Satan showed up and said…
Genesis 3:1 "Has God indeed said, 'You shall not eat of every tree of the garden'?

2 And the woman said to the serpent, "We may eat the fruit of the trees of the garden;

3 but of the fruit of the tree which is in the midst of the garden, God has said, 'You shall not eat it, nor shall you touch it, lest you die."

4 Then the serpent said to the woman, "You will not surely die.

5 For God knows that in the day you eat of it your eyes will be opened and you will be like God, **knowing good and evil."**

6 So when the woman saw that the tree was good for food, that it was pleasant to the eyes, and a tree desirable to make one wise, she took of its fruit and ate. She also gave to her husband with her, and he ate.

7 Then the eyes of both of them were opened, and they knew that they were naked; and they sewed fig leaves together and made themselves coverings."

So what really happened here that was so devastating to the human race that it caused us to spin out of control and down a path of destruction, sickness, disease, poverty and ultimately death?

The perfect law of belief was broken and they chose to believe in something else other than God!

Adam and Eve decided they didn't believe God when He said not to eat of the fruit of the tree of the knowledge of good and evil or they would die!

The minute Adam and Eve chose to eat of the tree of the knowledge of good and evil and chose to not believe God, they broke the core law that was absolutely critical to the harmony of all creation.

The law of believing God!

They and God became a house divided!

Mathew 25 But Jesus knew their thoughts, and said to them: "Every kingdom divided against itself is brought to desolation, and every city or house divided against itself will not stand.

But because our Creator already knew this would happen, He designed a plan to help us find our way back into fellowship & belief in Him.

His design is so perfect that if we are willing to believe Him, failure is impossible!

We can have the desires of our hearts as soon we are restored to Him.

Is God being cruel and causing us to suffer until He gets His way?

Absolutely not, we suffer because we broke our Creators "rules of construction (laws)" which causes severe malfunctions in the harmony of His perfect creation.

The result of this is chaos and confusion.

As in society whenever a law is broken a price has to be paid.

His amazing plan of restoration and redemption was to pay the price for breaking the law of belief in Him...through the sacrifice, death, burial and resurrection of His only Son Yeshua (Jesus)!

This is a debt or fine we couldn't pay ourselves so he paid it Himself to demonstrate to us the power of His Love!

John 3:16
For God so loved the world that He gave His only begotten Son, that whoever believes in Him should not perish but have everlasting life (the law of the Spirit of Life in Christ overriding the law of sin and death).

We all participate in the law of belief in one way or another, and just like all laws; the law of belief will work for us or against us, whether we understand it or not.

Because Adam & Eve disobeyed God and ate the fruit of the tree of the knowledge of good & evil, mankind suddenly got a conscience. We now all know when we do wrong or when we do right.

So when mankind moved from the higher law of life through unbelief and fell to the lower law of sin and death we also acquired a conscience (knowledge of good and evil).

Along with our conscience and separation from God came sickness, disease, poverty, lack and condemnation.

Condemnation is a killer!

Suddenly we were exposed to negative feelings and emotions, which have been scientifically proven to cause our physical bodies to break down and die.

So when we do wrong our conscience condemns us and this condemnation builds up over time, so much so that it causes us to fail in life, get sick, and many times die before our time.

1 John; 20 For if our heart condemns us, God is greater than our heart, and knows all things. 21 Beloved, if our heart does not condemn us, we have confidence toward God.

Scientifically what happens when we live under condemnation (negative emotions) is, our DNA constricts and our immune system shuts down.

We have been in prison under a sentence of death... until Jesus appeared and set us free by paying the price for breaking the Law of Belief.

He gave His Life to release us from the Law of Sin and Death.

He purchased life for us and obtained forgiveness and restored all who believe back to the fullness and fellowship that Yeshua (Jesus) has with God the Father.

By bearing every sin sickness & disease that ever existed past, present and future on Himself at the cross there is nothing left to pay if we dare to believe!

We are forgiven and restored to complete fullness, if we are willing to believe Him.

This includes healing, prosperity and fullness of life.

Forgiveness in the Strong's concordance means released from prison or bondage.

And so... because our Creator loved us so much, He gave His only begotten Son Jesus, to have us released from bondage and imprisonment under the Law of Sin and Death.

John 3:16 For God so loved the world that He gave His only begotten Son, that whoever believes in Him should not perish but have everlasting life.

By believing what He did we become new spirit at the core of our being and nothing (even if we fail) will separate from His Love & restoration.

Paul said in 1 Corinthians 38; For I am persuaded that neither death nor life, nor angels nor principalities nor powers, nor things present nor things to come, 39 nor height nor depth, nor any other created thing, shall be able to separate us from the love of God which is in Christ Jesus our Lord.

Jesus took our place and paid for the breaking of His laws in full, to restore us to the Law of Life in Christ Jesus, with all the privileges and benefits that come with it.

If we dare to believe!

The price Jesus paid gives us the absolute 100% right to be completely and fully restored to the Law of Life in Him, if we choose to receive and BELIEVE Him.

This means you and I have the right to live with the same abilities and fullness that Jesus had when He walked the earth!

But here's what many Christians have missed, that causes us to withdraw from Him.

We think when we fail to live up to Gods standard, He pushes us away.

We think in order to get back in His good graces we have to do good things and then He will accept us again.

The fact is, if we could get back into fellowship with Him by our good works, Jesus wouldn't have had to die to restore us!

The fact is, if we are in Christ, every failing (sin) past present and future is already paid for, so when we fail (sin), we can have complete confidence we are safe and secure in Him forever.

We don't run away from Him we can run to Him for help in overcoming our failings.

The GOOD NEWS is, no matter how many times we fail...today, tomorrow or next week Jesus paid once and for all, for every failing (sin) on the cross.

Does that mean we can live a life of sin, do whatever we want to do with no consequences?

If you WANT to sin, you haven't been delivered from the Law of Sin and Death!

That's right, if you are a truly born again and living under the Law of Life in Christ Jesus, you may fail and sin, but you don't want to sin. You will always do your best not to sin.

But if we do fail, the price has already been paid and we don't have to run away from Him.

He doesn't see our sins, because they are already paid for!

You may say to me...how can our Creator not see our sin when we fail, once we've accepted Jesus Christ?

In the Old Testament Numbers 28 Balak a King hired Balaam a prophet of God to curse the nation of Israel.

Long story short Balaam said this... Numbers 23 21 "He (God) has not observed iniquity in Jacob, Nor has He seen wickedness in Israel.

God couldn't see their sin!

How is this possible?

The sacrificial offerings for sin made by the Priests of God removed sin from Israel for a year.

God couldn't see their sin (failures) because of the blood of animals shed, to atone for the nations sin.

What does God see when He looks at you?

He sees Jesus.

Romans 8 There is therefore now no condemnation to those who are in Christ Jesus,

This truth will absolutely rock your world, shatter your preconceptions and place you squarely into health, prosperity and fullness of life!

Once we're in Christ Jesus...NOTHING can EVER EVER EVER separate us from Him!

Think about that...

He did it all and we did nothing but accept what He did for us and now we are entitled to live healthy, prosperous lives in this life and in the life to come, eternity.

Luke 18:29 So He said to them, "Assuredly, I say to you, there is no one who has left house or parents or brothers or wife or children, for the sake of the kingdom of God, 30 who shall not **receive many times more in this present time, and in the age to come eternal life.**"

We all believe something, and the good news is that we can change our beliefs at the very core of our being with His help!

Whether you believe you can or you believe you can't...you're right.

Everything in the quantum unseen world creates the physical makeup of what we see, hear, smell and experience in this physical seen world.

And remember, the most amazing thing about this discovery is that what we believe has been scientifically proven to alter or change things in the quantum/unseen world.

To put it another way... your thoughts and beliefs change you and the world around you for better or for worse depending on your belief system.

Here's some scripture to back up how powerful our beliefs are and how important it is to believe right!

Psalm 27:13 I would have lost heart, unless I had **believed** that I would see the goodness of the Lord In the land of the living.
Daniel 6:23 and no injury whatever was found on him, because he **believed** in his God.

Matthew 8:13 Then Jesus said to the centurion, "Go your way; and as you have **believed**, so let it be done for you."

Mark 5:36 As soon as Jesus heard the word that was spoken, He said to the ruler of the synagogue, "Do not be afraid; only **believe**.

Mark 9:23 Jesus said to him, "If you can **believe**, all things are possible to him who **believes**."

Mark 11:23 For assuredly, I say to you, whoever says to this mountain, 'Be removed and be cast into the sea,' and does not doubt in his heart, but **believes** that those things he says will be done, he will have whatever he says.

Mark 11:24 Therefore I say to you, whatever things you ask when you pray, **believe** that you receive them, and you will have them.

Mark 16: He who **believes** and is baptized will be saved; but he who **does not believe** will be condemned.

Mark 16:17 And these signs will follow those who **believe**: In My name they will cast out demons; they will speak with new tongues;

Luke 1:45 Blessed is she who **believed**, for there will be a fulfillment of those things which were told her from the Lord."

Luke 8:12 Those by the wayside are the ones who hear; then the devil comes and takes away the word out of their hearts, lest they should **believe** and be saved.

Luke 8:50 But when Jesus heard it, He answered him, saying, "Do not be afraid; only **believe**, and she will be made well."

John 1:12 But as many as received Him, to them He gave the right to become children of God, to those who **believe** in His name:

John 3:15 that whoever **believes** in Him should not perish but have eternal life.

John 3:16 For God so loved the world that He gave His only begotten Son, that whoever **believes** in Him should not perish but have everlasting life.

John 3:18 "He who **believes** in Him is not condemned; but he who does not believe is condemned already, because he has not believed in the name of the only begotten Son of God.

John 3:36 He who **believes** in the Son has everlasting life; and he who does not believe the Son shall not see life, but the wrath of God abides on him."
John 6:29 Jesus answered and said to them, "This is the work of God, that you **believe** in Him whom He sent."

John 6:35 And Jesus said to them, "I am the bread of life. He who comes to Me shall never hunger, and he who **believes** in Me shall never thirst.

John 6:40 And this is the will of Him who sent Me, that everyone who sees the Son and **believes** in Him may have everlasting life; and I will raise him up at the last day."

John 12:36 While you have the light, **believe** in the light, that you may become sons of light."

John 14:12 "Most assuredly, I say to you, he who **believes** in Me, the works that I do he will do also; and greater works than these he will do, because I go to My Father.

Let me recommend a book to you that I study over and over to help me change my core beliefs… in fact this author/preachers writings/teachings can literally change your life forever.

The book is called **The Power of Right Believing by Joseph Prince**. If you're serious about changing your belief system Joseph's ministry will change your life!

Chapter 9

Why Miracles Work for Some and Not for Others

So why do some people get a miracle while others don't?

To answer that question we need to go to the very heart of how the Creation was flawlessly designed from the very beginning.

Let's dig a little deeper...

This is where I may step on some toes, but what I'm about to share with you, has the power to change your life forever!

The Bible says that there is an unpardonable sin. The scripture I'm referring to is Mark 3:28

28 "Assuredly, I say to you, all sins will be forgiven the sons of men, and whatever blasphemies they may utter;

29 but he who blasphemes against the Holy Spirit never has forgiveness, but is subject to eternal condemnation"—

30 because they said, "He has an unclean spirit."

At first glance you would think that the unpardonable sin is when someone curses or rails against the Holy Spirit of God.

But let's back up a little and put this into context. This is what was going on before Jesus brought up the unpardonable sin

A House Divided Cannot Stand

22 And the scribes who came down from Jerusalem said, "He has Beelzebub," and, "By the ruler of the demons He casts out demons."

23 So He called them to Himself and said to them in parables: "How can Satan cast out Satan?

24 If a kingdom is divided against itself, that kingdom cannot stand.

25 And if a house is divided against itself, that house cannot stand.

26 And if Satan has risen up against himself, and is divided, he cannot stand, but has an end.

Do you see it?

The scribes are railing against Jesus who represents the Holy Spirit of God, because **they don't believe Him.**

And if they don't believe Him... they and He are a house divided.

If they don't believe Him, but want to be part of His Kingdom, the Kingdom of God would become a house divided and couldn't stand! Therefore the unpardonable sin is not believing God.

This is exactly the same problem that occurred in the Garden of Eden.

We're back to square one!

God can't forgive or pardon us when we choose to believe in something other than Him... because then He would be ruler of a divided Kingdom and it wouldn't last.

It's not because He doesn't love us or want to forgive us... but if we don't believe Him... there's nothing He can do for us.

It's our choice!

How can we live in harmony inside His creation... when we don't believe the Creator?

We can't!

Look around you... the world as we know it today... is a house divided and therefore, it has an end just as the Bible declares.

Does this mean that we won't make it to the heavenly kingdom because there are some things we are having trouble believing?
Absolutely not, Jesus Himself said in John 6:40
"And this is the will of Him who sent Me, that everyone who sees the Son and believes in Him may have everlasting life; and I will raise him up at the last day."

Let me make this clear... as long as you believe that Jesus Christ is the Son of God, and that He died to forgive you of your sins... and you've asked His forgiveness, and made Him your Lord & Saviour... you have eternal life with Him!

Romans 10:9 that if you confess with your mouth the Lord Jesus and believe in your heart that God has raised Him from the dead, you will be saved.

But because life is a growth process, if we aren't living in the fullness that God has provided for us right now, and we want to be, we will need to develop our belief system to a deeper level.

None of the disciples got everything right all at once; they were in a growth process right up until they left the earth.

But we know because every disciple exept John died a martyr's death, they certainly believed!

Let's go deeper.

Matthew 21:22
And whatever things you ask in prayer, believing, you will receive."

Do you believe at the very core of your being, in your heart of hearts, that the miracle you are seeking will manifest itself in this physical realm?

Can you visualize yourself living in your miracle and feel the emotions you would have, as if it's already happened?

Do you really believe that God meets all your need according to His riches in glory by Christ Jesus?

If you can your miracle is on the way!

If you can't don't be alarmed!

You've identified the area you need to work on, and you can start by changing your belief system in your heart of hearts, using the techniques provided in the following chapters.

As we have learned, the study of Quantum Physics proves that what we believe or what we don't believe, manifests in our lives for good or for bad.

If you are a Christian, the Bible tells us that through Jesus... we have been restored to the Law of Life in Him, to live full healthy abundant lives NOW and in the life to come.

But that's just the tip of the iceberg... He even told us that we would do greater things than He did!

Coming from Someone who walked on water, raised the dead and healed the sick, that means to me that we have the abilities to do what He did and more, if our belief system is functioning at its highest level.

If we aren't living full healthy abundant lives, and if we aren't living in the miraculous the way we want to don't panic.

Our belief system is flawed and simply needs some work.

The Bible also says you shall know the truth, and the truth will set you free.

Truth can be a hard pill to swallow, especially when it's truth about us.

The good news is, if we don't get offended, we can achieve victory and success beyond our wildest dreams.

If we're not afraid to look at ourselves and work on the areas in our lives that need change, we can live in the miraculous forever.

The Bible and science are merging at such an incredibly accelerated pace, that it's getting easier and easier for us to comprehend, understand and believe our Creator.

Everything in creation was designed to work in complete harmony with everything else through His perfect system of laws.

Through a deeper understanding of our Creators system of laws, we are now able prove beyond a shadow of a doubt the truth of His Word.

One of the most powerful versus in the Bible that reveals how the Law of Belief functions at the quantum level is this one.

Hebrews Chapter 11 vs. 1 & 3

Faith is the substance of things hoped for the evidence of things not seen

When I looked into the root of the above words I found that you could also say it like this...

Belief is the foundation in full confidence, the proof of that which has been done (an accomplished fact), not seen by the naked eye...

... By Faith we understand that the worlds were framed by the Word of God so that the things which are seen (Newtonian Physics) were not made of things which are visible (Quantum Physics).

Chapter 10

The Creation Process

When we truly believe something in our heart/core... when something in us BELIEVES sees and feels it coming to pass in our minds eye, before it manifests itself in this physical realm, we are in the creation process at the quantum level.

The same way our Creator made the creation.
God says we are made in His image.
Genesis 1:26

Then God said, "Let Us make man in Our image, according to Our likeness;

We have been given creative power at the very core of our being, to bring events to pass in our lives that may not be seen in the physical world YET.

Every probable outcome to every situation has already been placed within the grasp of each one of us.

All we have to do is pick the outcome we want, believe in our hearts it will come to pass, and all the other probable outcomes will collapse... leaving only the one we choose to believe.

If we are sick or broke, it's because our belief system is flawed at the core of our being, and we have trouble seeing ourselves as healthy and prosperous.

The Law of Belief isn't functioning to its highest level in our lives yet.

But the Gospel (Good News) is that we can have any Godly desire now in this life if we dare to believe...and in the Life to come!

Jesus wasn't into stuff and yet whatever He wanted... was provided for.

He was a Man of miracles and we are told to do as He did.

One time Peter asked Jesus about paying temple taxes.

Mathew 17: 27 nevertheless, lest we offend them, go to the sea, cast in a hook, and take the fish that comes up first.

And when you have opened its mouth, you will find a piece of money; take that and give it to them for me and you."

Jesus was a man living in a mortal body like you and I except He was a perfect man without sin.

He had to walk the earth under the same laws that we live under in order to show us how to live, and to encourage us that we could do what He asked of us.

Therefore he couldn't operate in any more power than what is also available to us, or we couldn't possibly do what He expects from us.

How did He do this amazing miracle?

I'm fully persuaded that at the quantum level, He visualized and felt the emotions of the outcome He wanted, and believed in His heart that it would come to pass, and the result manifested in this world just as He knew it would!

Jesus belief in His Father was so developed and profound that it was easy for Him.

The stronger we develop our belief in God the easier it will be to bring miracles to pass on our lives and the lives of those around us.

Jesus said in Matthew 21:22 "And whatever things you ask in prayer, believing, you will receive".

Let's look at what He said was possible for us to do.

Mark 11:23
For assuredly, I say to you, whoever says to this mountain, 'Be removed and be cast into the sea,' and does not doubt in his heart, but believes that those things he says will be done, he will have whatever he says.

The facts are irrefutable... all we have to do is believe what God says... in our hearts and we will have whatever we ask for.

Mark 9:23 Jesus said to him, "If you can believe, all things are possible to him who believes."

The good news according to the Law of Belief and Quantum Physics is... if we change what we believe on the inside of us at the quantum level... our beliefs will change us and the world around us.

We all have God given creative power inside us, to get a miracle for our healing, for our prosperity or for any Godly desire we can think of!

So how do we do this? How do we change at the heart level?

When Jesus hung on that horrible cross for us... He looked up to heaven and said... "It is finished."

I believe that this means exactly what He said...
IT IS FINISHED. There was nothing left for God
to do; now it's up to us!

Chapter 11

The Miracle is in You

Our Creator has put into our hands right now...
everything we need to walk in the absolute
fullness that He originally intended for us to
walk in even though we are still living inside our
mortal corruptible body.

Everything is available to us right now in this
life... and the life to come! It's all in His Word!

Dare to Believe!

When we receive the sacrifice Jesus paid to
restore us to Him, we instantly become a new
creation (spirit) in our core being.

2 Corinthians 5: 17 Therefore, if anyone is in
Christ, he is a new creation; old things have
passed away; behold all things have become new.

**The Creator of the universe literally
comes to live in us.**

Galatians 2:20 I have been crucified with Christ; it is no longer I who live, but Christ lives in me; and the life which I now live in the flesh I live by faith in the Son of God, who loved me and gave Himself for me.

Colossians 1:27 Christ in you, the hope of glory.

He is the miracle in us!

Does that mean we live our lives with no failures?

No we are still in this corruptible body until the body dies.

Our job is to feed our new spirit until it becomes stronger than our corruptible flesh, **but if we fail, the price has already been paid and there are no more penalties or condemnation**...we are FREE!

John 8:36 Therefore if the Son makes you free, you shall be free indeed.

So the next step for us is to learn to live in the miraculous.

Chapter 12

You Are the Creator of Your Destiny

We all have the freedom to choose how to live our lives and our choices are a direct result of what we truly believe deep in our core being.

If we believe there is lack, then for us there is lack because either we don't believe what our Creator says or, we don't know the promises He has given to us.

Let me explain.

If you took a cruise where everything was provided, but didn't know the food and drinks were free, you might bring food and eat it in your cabin, instead of eating and drinking the banquet provided for free.

Only because you didn't know what was available for you!

It pays to know what is yours, that's why I study Gods Word, I don't want to miss out on anything!

Philippians 4:19 And my God shall supply all your need according to His riches in glory by Christ Jesus.

Do you believe Him?

In His word He has made it very clear what is needed to live full abundant lives here and now and what is required to be accepted into His eternal Kingdom.

Hebrews Chapter 11 vs. 6 says

For without Faith (Belief) it is impossible to please God for he who comes to God must BELIEVE that He is... and that he rewards those who diligently seek Him

He also says in His Word, that His eye searches throughout the earth to perform His Word

If we trust God, and believe what He says is true and act on it, then the Law of Belief He has set in motion will create health, abundance and purpose for us.

But that's just the beginning!

As we grow in our belief in Him, we will walk down the same path that Jesus walked... and we will live our entire lives inside the realm of the miraculous.

Mark 11:24 Therefore I say to you, whatever things you ask when you pray, believe that you receive them, and you will have them.

He doesn't need to supernaturally intervene to get us healed or make us prosperous... it's already done... if we dare to believe!

We have been given everything needed for rich full abundant life.

One of the incredible tools God has given us to know if we are on the right path, is our feelings and emotions.

We can pinpoint exactly where we stand with laser accuracy, by monitoring the feelings and emotions we have around the issues in our lives.

For example, are you afraid you'll lose your job or not have enough money to pay the bills?

Then that's simply an area of your belief system that needs to be built up.

Feelings and emotions are the keys to finding out what is good for us and what isn't.

By training ourselves to consciously monitor our feelings and emotions as we go through our day...we will begin to understand and uncover what we need to change in our daily lives in order to live in the miraculous.

When you look at it this way, it really becomes simple to begin changing what is hurting us and doing more of what is good for us!

And because we are working with laws, they will never fail.

Chapter 13

Love or Fear… What's Controlling Your Life?

There are two major emotions… love (positive) and fear (negative)… out of which flow all other positive or negative emotions.

John 4:18 There is no fear in love; but perfect love casts out fear, because fear involves torment. But he who fears has not been made perfect in love.

1 John 4:8 He who does not love does not know God, for God is love.

Here God is telling us in words how things work at the quantum level without getting into details.

The more we walk in love the more we live the way we were created to live!

The more we live in fear or negative emotions the more we live apart from His Way.

Scientifically it has been proven that when we are feeling fear, hate... or any negative emotions that come out of fear... our DNA constricts and our immune system shuts down.

It has also been proven scientifically that when we are feeling love peace and joy or any other positive emotions that come from love, our DNA relaxes and our immune system flourishes.

In one experiment scientists recruited people who were trained to give off emotions on demand and isolated their DNA.

These people could instantly turn on the emotions of love, appreciation and compassion or fear, anger and hate.

They could literally have those feelings and emotions on demand.

This means the we can learn to do the same thing!

The test subjects along with their DNA were wired up to bio feedback equipment that could monitor their DNA.

What they discovered was... that when the test subjects gave off emotions of love, appreciation and compassion, their DNA relaxed and their immune system flourished.

When they gave off emotions of hate, anger, fear or rage, their DNA constricted and their immune system shut down.

If we are in a health or financial crisis... and we feed our spirit a diet of negative energy such as fear or stress... the results will be disastrous!

The Bible consistently exhorts us to "Fear Not."

Isaiah 41:10
Fear not, for I am with you; Be not dismayed, for I am your God. I will strengthen you, Yes, I will help you, I will uphold you with My righteous right hand.'

Isaiah 44:2
Thus says the LORD who made you and formed you from the womb, who will help you: '**Fear not**

Quantum Physics is revealing to us scientifically, that the Law of Fear... when in operation in our lives causes us great harm.

If we are feeding ourselves a steady diet of love and peace or any positive emotion the Law of Love takes over... our DNA relaxes and our immune system flourishes.

Chapter 14

Harnessing The Power of Emotions

In order to get a miracle it is necessary to combine the right belief system along with the right feelings and emotions that are needed to generate a change in your life at the quantum level.

Quantum Physicist Doctor John Hagelin PHD says that **our body is really the product of our thoughts and emotions**.

He goes on to explain; "We're beginning to understand in Medical Science the degree to which the nature of thoughts and emotions actually determines the physical substance and structure and function of our bodies"

Do you really know what you believe in your heart?

I myself didn't know my true beliefs until I went through a very hard time in my life.

Then I saw a critical area in me, that needed to change, but I didn't know how to change my beliefs down at the core of my being.

What I'm sharing with you are the results that came to me through intensive research that was driven by much pain and sorrow.

To truly change at the core of our being we must be brutally honest with ourselves and look at the results of our lives.

That is if we really want to change

Jesus said... Luke 6:44 "For every tree is known by its own fruit"

How's your fruit?

Is your life truly filled with joy, health and abundance?

If it isn't, then find out what heart/core beliefs you need to change and change them!

Train yourself to become aware of your feelings and emotions at all times no matter where you are or what you are doing.

When we notice our feelings and emotions are negative (fear based) we need to immediately stop what we are doing and practice giving off the positive emotions of love, peace, and joy to replace our negative emotions.

It's as simple as completely stopping whatever activity is causing these negative feelings and emotions.

Then replace that activity with one that generates the feelings and emotions that are love based and positive.

The point I'm making here is, monitor your feelings and emotions and when they go negative, stop the activity.

Listen very closely to your feelings and emotions at all times and trust that as you learn to manage them, you'll be literally changing the vibrational tone of your energy at the quantum level!

And, according to Quantum Physics will bring about change in your physical body and surroundings.

This will require effort and if your desire is strong you will succeed!

At first it may seem hard, but it gets much easier the more you practice.

Eventually it will become automatic.

When you learned to tie your shoes, it was hard at first... but suddenly you didn't even think about it, you just did it.

As our belief system along with our feelings and emotions, begin to line up with God's perfect will for us... suddenly our health will spring forth and any lack that is in our lives will become filled to overflowing.

Chapter 15

Changing Our Core Beliefs

It's important to note here that if you received Jesus as your Lord and Saviour you literally become a new creature!

2 Corinthians 5:17
Therefore, if anyone is in Christ, he is a new creation; old things have passed away; behold, all things have become new.

The problem is that our bodies and old thinking processes are still there and are constantly trying to override our new baby spirit.

Changing your core belief system (old man) will initially seem very hard at first but we want to change our belief patterns, in such a way that our new beliefs become automatic and we don't even think about them anymore.

Remember...the patterns that we've developed over our entire life have become firmly rooted in our sub-conscious.

It's important that you have a basic understanding of the process involved in changing your beliefs at the heart level.

It has been said that our conscious mind operates at only 5% of our entire mind function.

The majority of our mind operates at the sub-conscious level.

In order to change our core belief system, we will need to change at the sub-conscious level.

Don't worry this simply involves setting up new habits that will become second nature after practice.

And remember... we're learning how to live in the miraculous... but this does require a strong desire on our part!

The sub-conscious mind operates something like this.

Imagine yourself driving a car while talking with a passenger. You don't have to focus on the route, the stops or your surroundings, to drive safely to your destination.

Your sub-conscious mind is easily managing all these things for you, while your conscious mind is talking with your passenger.

To change our core beliefs we have to re-program ourselves at the subconscious level... so that living in the miraculous will become second nature and automatic.

During the ages of 0-6 our brains recorded and interpreted how the world works, and set in motion what we believed our place and abilities in the world were.

We formed the foundation of what we believed it was possible for us to do in life at that very early age.

We learned our current belief system from our interactions with our family and the environment around us.

Right or wrong these patterns were ingrained into our core beings at the sub conscious level and we have been living from these beliefs ever since.

Everything we listen to, read, and watch on TV and even the people that are around us, all reinforce our belief system, which ultimately rules our lives.

Many times when people attend self-help seminars and get back home ready to apply this new found knowledge, nothing changes.

This is because we are only using the conscious 5% level of our brains without knowing how to move these new ideas into the core of our being at the sub conscious level.

We come home from a seminar and we're ready to change but the minute our conscious mind becomes distracted and we start to focus on life in general our old sub-conscious patterns take over once again.

Then we look around and say...that stuff I learned at the seminar doesn't work.

And that's the end of it.

To live in the miraculous we need to have our entire being at the very core subconscious level, working for our good all the time not just when we are thinking about it.

We do this by changing our beliefs at the sub-conscious level.

When we put these new concepts into our belief system at the sub conscious level we put them into practice on auto pilot

Chapter 16

Meditation and Visualization the Secret Power of Miracles

We can change and strengthen our core heart beliefs through proven age old methods used by many different groups of people for centuries.

In order to master these techniques and use them to live the way our Creator intended, it's critical that we are not afraid to think outside the box, and that we work with Truth no matter where we find it.

The Bible comes from the Middle East from a people who don't think like we think in western civilization.

Meditation was a way of life and the Bible is full of meditation and visualization.

Here's some scripture to back this up.

Genesis 24:63 And Isaac went out to **meditate** in the field in the evening

Joshua 1:8 This Book of the Law shall not depart from your mouth, but you shall **meditate** in it day and night, that you may observe to do according to all that is written in it.

Psalm 1:2 But his delight is in the law of the Lord, And in His law he **meditates** day and night.

Psalm 4:4 Be angry, and do not sin. **Meditate** within your heart on your bed, and be still. Selah

Psalm 63:6 When I remember You on my bed, I **meditate** on You in the night watches.

Psalm 77:6 I call to remembrance my song in the night; I **meditate** within my heart, and my spirit makes diligent search.

Psalm 119:15 I will **meditate** on Your precepts, And contemplate Your ways

Psalm 119:23 Princes also sit and speak against me, But Your servant **meditates** on Your statutes.

Remember most of the people in the Bible didn't know how to read or write. There weren't books or any of the convenient ways we have of learning today.

Many of the teachers of the Torah (Old Testament) memorized it word for word and could quote it on demand.

Passing these events down from generation to generation by parchment and word of mouth was the way it was done.

Families would sit together and the scriptures would be recited while the people literally visualized, pondered and meditated on them.

In Joshua 1:8 the Creator said "This Book of the Law shall not depart from your mouth, but you shall **meditate** in it day and night, that you may observe to do according to all that is written in it. For then you will make your way prosperous, and then you will have good success.

The word meditate, in the Strong's concordance means 1) to roar, growl, groan 2) to **utter, speak** 3) to meditate, devise, muse, **imagine**.

Imagine...

What we imagine or visually see ourselves doing in our minds physiologically generates a response in our bodies as if we were really actually there doing the event.

This act causes changes deep within us at the quantum level.

Visualize yourself living the life you want and combine the emotions of how you would feel while living that life.

If you are having problems with your health see and feel how it would be living without your disability.

The same goes when you read your Bible, read it out loud and personalize it.

As we visualize ourselves right there watching & participating in what was going on, we strengthen our belief and trust in God while we imprint Truth on the inward part of us.

When we visualize and actually feel ourselves swimming, running or walking when we are laying in our bed unable to rise, will start things moving in that direction at the quantum level.

Remember energy flows where attention goes.

The art of meditation is something that we need to study, learn and implement into our lives on a daily basis.

The more we believe and trust God, the easier it is for us to live in the miraculous just like Jesus did.

Cathy Goodman, the lady who was healed of breast cancer consciously and deliberately removed all stress from her life.

She watched funny videos and laughed all the time.

According to Scientific American... "When laughter is elicited, pain thresholds are significantly increased, whereas when subjects watched something that does not naturally elicit laughter, pain thresholds do not change (and are often lower)," the authors write in the paper.

"These results can best be explained by the action of endorphins released by laughter."

The Bible verse to back that up is Proverbs 17:22 A merry heart does good, like medicine, But a broken spirit dries the bones.

She visualized herself as already healed not going to be healed, and adopted a posture of gratefulness!

Visualization has been scientifically proven to alter the physical results of the body.

"In one of the most well-known studies on creative visualization in sports, Russian scientists compared four groups of Olympic athletes in terms of their physical and mental training ratios:

• Group 1 received 100% physical training;
• Group 2 received 75% physical training with 25% mental training;
• Group 3 received 50% mental training with 50% physical training;
• Group 4 received 75% mental training with 25% physical training.

Group 4 had the best performance results, indicating that certain types of mental training, such as consciously invoking specific subjective states, can have significant measurable effects on biological performance.

According to Cummins,

The Soviets had discovered that mental images (imaginations) can act as a prelude to muscular impulses

It has since become more widely understood and accepted in neuroscience and sports psychology that subjective training can cause the body to respond more favorably to consciously desired outcomes".

Chapter 17

The Law of Gratitude

Philippians 4 vs. 4 says to rejoice in the Lord always and again I say rejoice!

Something happens deep within our hearts when we maintain a constant state of gratitude and thankfulness and rejoicing.

We were created to live this way!

As Cathy Goodman, the woman healed from breast cancer went through her ordeal; she constantly kept herself in a state of gratefulness and thanked God for her healing as if it had already happened.

When we become truly grateful it's impossible to remain negative and fearful. We literally accelerate our ability to live in the miraculous.

By doing this Cathy relaxed her DNA and her immune system flourished and did what it was designed to do, heal her body.

Zoologist Frank Sherwin points out that there are proteins called Editase that move over our DNA and monitor and replace mistakes in our DNA on a second by second, minute by minute time frame.

Negative emotions literally kill this process of healing and correction.

As mentioned, when we are on the love side of our feelings and emotions, it has been proven our DNA functions at its optimum level.

Did you know that physically our bodies replace and rebuild themselves every couple of years? Some parts of our bodies are replaced every second.

It is critical to our health and prosperity that we keep our emotions on the positive emotion side as much as possible, while our cellular structure replaces itself.

It's critical to our success and health that we consistently visualize and feel the feelings of what we want right now in the present.

By doing this we take control of our future and start moving toward the destiny that we were meant to live.

We are not in denial that we need health or prosperity; we are simply causing our body, through the creative process at the quantum level, to begin to move in the right direction.

Way-FM

One of the most important tools I use to keep my emotions supercharged and focused on the positive, is my daily listening to Way-FM (wayfm.com)

Honestly I don't know what I'd do without this national radio station.

Wally and his team have the morning show and they do a fantastic job keeping the energy positive... as does everyone over at Way-FM

Way-FM radio is syndicated across the United States but you can listen from anywhere in the world with the Way FM app for Android or iPhone.

Tune in I guarantee it will change your life!

Chapter 18

Meditation Secrets

Here's an example of how to practice Godly biblical meditation that will help you believe in a deeper way, while replacing other beliefs that have been holding you back from living life in the miraculous.

The more you do this the faster you will get your miracle.

You will learn what it is to live in a state of being where you have no fear and the more victories you have the easier and easier this will be for you.

The best time to meditate is when you first wake up in the morning before the cares and worries of the day set in.

You will need to allow yourself at least an hour for this...

Here's a tip that I use and it has never failed me! I allow myself the luxury of drinking two cups of coffee during this time. I even setup the coffee maker next to my bed, load it with coffee and water and set the timer to go off when I want to wake up.

Instead of waking up to a jarring noisy alarm, I hear the coffee maker go off. I know I still have to wait for it, so I stay in that peaceful state of being.

We are in our most suggestible state when we are between waking and sleep.

While the coffee is perking, I consciously practice feeling the emotions of peace, joy and gratefulness by focusing my attention on the good things in my life.

Things like the simple pleasures of having a comfortable bed to sleep in and a roof over my head to keep out the weather.

I imagine myself laughing, which has been scientifically proven to release endorphins, even while physically I'm not actually laughing.

Then when the coffee is ready, I prop up the pillows, pour a cup and open my Bible to whatever passage I decide to meditate on.

Now what I'm going to say next is critical. Don't have a goal of finishing a certain number of verses or getting into a competition with yourself.

Don't worry how much you did or didn't read the day before!

This is a new day.

You want the scriptures to minister to you at the deepest level possible... so you may just read and ponder a verse, or you may read the whole chapter.

The point is, flow with it. Always read it audibly softly or loudly, it's up to you, but read it out loud.

By doing this you will begin to strengthen your belief or faith at the core of your being, in your heart of hearts.

Remember one definition of meditation was to mutter or utter.

As you meditate, think of it as if you are pumping iron at the gym, the more you do this the stronger your belief system becomes.

As you sip your coffee, read a verse out loud and ponder upon it.

Romans 10:17 So then faith comes by hearing, and hearing by the word of God.

As you read out loud visualize yourself as being right there at that time in history, smell the smells, imagine what would be going on around you.

Say the verse again, sip the coffee, meditate some more and then move ahead and let the story unfold before your eyes.

Take your time!

If I'm going through a battle of my own, whether its health or finances or something that is very serious to me, one of the main weapons I meditate from is Hebrews 11 and even into 12.

Verse 32-34 is particularly powerful for me!

32 And what more shall I say? For the time would fail me to tell of Gideon and Barak and Samson and Jephthah, also of David and Samuel and the prophets:

33 who through faith subdued kingdoms, worked righteousness, obtained promises, stopped the mouths of lions,

34 quenched the violence of fire, escaped the edge of the sword, out of weakness were made strong, became valiant in battle, turned to flight the armies of the aliens.

who through faith subdued kingdoms...

Say the above scripture a few times out loud.

who through faith subdued kingdoms...

who through faith subdued kingdoms...

King David and many others subdued kingdoms through faith in God.

I visualize myself living fighting alongside King David and I practice radiating feelings of complete confidence that we have already won the battle.

I imagine and feel the power of God radiating out of me, as I visualize myself meeting with King David and his generals after they had won a great victory against impossible odds.

I see them rejoicing and praising God. I join with them and feel the overwhelming joy they must have felt.

I repeat the above verse over and over again and let my mind take me over the battlefields of old where victory looked impossible but through faith in God, victory was accomplished.

I meditate on the time that Joshua and his army surrounded Jericho and visually watch the walls come down.

I imagine the awe that the Israelites must have felt as this miracle came to pass before their very eyes.

I rejoice in the miracle that God gifted to His believers through the law of belief. I imagine how it must have felt to be there when all of this was happening.

I feel the emotions of victory and let these emotions wash over me again and again.

Then while the emotions are still fresh and washing over me, I focus on a promise in the Bible that I'm believing God for, concerning me and what I need a miracle for.

For example if I need healing in my body I meditate on the verse "By His stripes I am healed" while the emotions of victory and success through God's promises continue to wash over my being.

I take communion every morning while I meditate on Jesus and what He did for me.

Get yourself a small portable communion set and keep it by your bedside and as you partake focus and see Jesus on the cross bearing your sickness, poverty or distress so you wouldn't have to.

See your sickness or poverty on Him while His health and abundance are transferred to you!

See Him as He is now sitting at the right hand of our Heavenly Father. 1 John 4:17...because as He is, so are we in this world.

Communion is a very powerful vehicle for magnifying His Spirit and manifesting His presence almost instantly.

His tangible Presence comes into the room every time I take communion and ministers to me.

I visualize myself as if the sickness never existed in my body and I see and feel myself doing the things that I would be doing as if I were completely healthy.

By doing this I strengthen my trust and belief in God at the very core of my being, and set in motion the creative power of faith and trust in God and his promises.

Now you try.

Move to the next passage in the verse.

Take a few deep breaths and visualize yourself with Daniel as his faith...

stopped the mouths of lions,

See yourself with Daniel in the lion's den.

See the powerful lions moving all around you and feel the energy, confidence and Power of the Holy Spirit radiating out of you.

Watch in awe and wonder at the magnificence of these creatures, while your faith and trust in God grows deep within you and stops the lions from tearing you to pieces.

Can you see it?

Can you feel it?

Then as you continue to feel and radiate the emotions from being victorious in the lion's den... see yourself victorious over whatever is coming against you in your life.

Visualize whatever is coming against you as if it was already defeated and see and feel yourself doing the things that you will do to celebrate the victory.

Are you beginning to see how this works?

Let's do another one...

Take more deep breaths and visualize yourself being thrown into a massive raging fiery furnace.

See yourself inside the fiery furnace with Shadrach Meshach and Abednego. Experience their faith as it...

quenches the violence of fire

Feel the emotions and excitement you would feel as you walk around the fiery furnace unharmed.

Look with amazement at your hands and feet while the flames swirl around you.

Continue this exercise for as long as you like, following down these verses in this passage, one by one... (who through belief)

- escaped the edge of the sword,
- out of weakness were made strong,
- became valiant in battle,
- turned to flight the armies of the aliens,
- Women received their dead raised to life again

Chapter 19

The Power Within You

Every one of us at this present moment... is the result of our past beliefs and the decisions that we've made up to this moment in time.

The good news is, as we learn to alter our state of being, and begin generating feelings and emotions of peace, love and gratefulness, we start to move ourselves into an entirely new reality, and harmonize ourselves with our Creator and His Law of Life.

By changing our fear based negative belief system to a love based positive belief system, we directly influence our future success in all areas of our lives.

Our focus in life should be to live, breathe and have our beings entirely operating inside the Law of Life.

This activates God's laws for our blessing and we will begin to manifest total abundance and health.

Don't try to figure out how your miracle will happen, it's Gods good pleasure to bring it to pass.

Simply harmonize your beliefs with Truth and visualize the health or abundance that is yours through our Creators perfect provision.

And let your miracle unfold before your very eyes!

Always remember to close your eyes for a period of time each day and visualize, feel and project the emotions you would have if you were totally healthy and living the lifestyle that you want.

Visualize yourself and FEEL THE EMOTIONS as if you were living that way right now in the present.

Set specific goals for this event to happen and make those goals realistic.

As the creative power within you grows, the time it takes to bring a miracle to pass in this physical realm from the quantum level will get shorter and shorter.

Chapter 20

Dare To Believe

Jesus was able to generate miracles instantaneously on demand and He said in John 14:14 If you ask anything in My name, I will do it.

Jesus raised the dead...walked on water...had gold retrieved from the mouth of a fish.

The Bible declares that Jesus was a perfect man without sin and He was subject to the same laws that we are.

He was showing us what was possible by operating on the right side of the Law of Belief and believing our Heavenly Father with all our being.

I can see Him meditating; visualizing, feeling and believing what He wanted to come to pass as if it was already accomplished.

Then what He chose to happen materialized in this physical world from the quantum unseen realm.

He told us we can do the same!

Consciously do things that bring you joy and happiness and avoid things that give you fear and stress.

For example debt is one of the major causes of sickness, disease, and a major killer of good relationships on global proportions!

Proverbs 22:7 The rich rules over the poor, And the borrower is servant to the lender.

It's time to be released from the bondage of debt no matter what you have to do.

Set up a debt reduction system and then meditate and visualize yourself living feeling and experiencing the life you truly want as if you were already living it.

Spend as much time as possible meditating and visualizing yourself leading a healthy prosperous life.

Watch and be alert for opportunities!

When opportunity presents itself... grab it and keep moving ahead. Don't let fear keep you back any more!

Consciously do whatever it takes to remove negative emotions every day.

Stop participating in any activity that causes you to give off negative emotions

This may seem like a lot of work, but if you are in a life and death situation or you are in serious financial trouble, you must do everything possible to live the positive emotions of Love (Law of Life) and stop participating in the Law of Fear (Sin and Death).

Chapter 21

Persistence Pays Big Dividends

Read this book and get the recorded audio version. Play it over and over again.

After a while your old toxic beliefs, feelings and emotions will be replaced with positive beliefs, feelings and emotions.

Then, you will start having more and more good things happen to you... while the bad things will begin to fall away.

Like a snowball rolling down a hill and gathering momentum, health and prosperity will increase in your life and the miraculous will become a way of life for you, as you re-arrange your belief system at the subconscious level.

Yes, this may seem impossible at first but as you begin using the visualization and meditation techniques this will start to happen for you.

If your family members or your spouse are causing great stress in your life, make a list of all the good things about them: change your focus from the negative things they do.

You can't change another person's belief system but you can change your beliefs about that person.

This will start to generate good emotions and start to shift your negative beliefs about that person.

Remember our Creator created everyone, and he loves everyone the same... which means everyone has the same opportunities to be healthy and prosperous and live full abundant lives.

Make a list of everything you are grateful for... and add to that list every time you think of something.

Whenever you are feeling down and negative pull out your "grateful list" and read it over... even add to it.

By doing this you will start to cause a shift in your belief patterns.

3: **Visualize and Meditate on what you want:**

If you need healing in your body then every day, several times a day become quiet, close your eyes, see and feel yourself perfectly healthy. You are not denying your infirmity or your lack of prosperity you are focusing your attention and your creative power on what you want to manifest in this physical realm.

You are literally imprinting what you want into your core being... which will bring it to pass in the physical world.

See and feel the way you would be as if sickness or disease was never in your body.

See and feel yourself living the lifestyle that you want for yourself and your family.

Live in that moment as if it was right now.

4: **Earnestly Repeat This Every Day:**

When I say every day that's just a guideline. If you want results faster visualize and meditate several times every day own what you want make it yours.

Chapter 23

How To Get Quicker Results

Watch videos, listen to audios and read books that strengthen your belief in God and use all your extra time meditating and visualizing what you want.

Always smile and watch your body language. Correct it when you find yourself assuming any posture that reflects fear or doubt and this will help your overall attitude.

Find a partner and work together to help each other.

BREATHE!

Watch your breathing at all times!

Breathe deeply and slowly. Your breathing is your body's regulator and if you catch yourself breathing short shallow breaths... your body will go into worry or panic mode.

Many people unconsciously will start to breathe short shallow quick breaths when they are in public without even knowing they are doing this. Watch funny videos and laugh every chance you get.

Praise and be thankful always!

This helps keep you develop a positive mental attitude.

Constantly remind yourself that there is One greater than us all, who loves us and has set in motion everything we would ever need to live healthy, prosperous abundant lives.

BONUS!

I have bonus material to help you that is available for you free of charge on the bonus page of my website! www.howtogetamiracle.com

I've added movies and music that you can watch anytime for free that will help you keep your focus when you need an entertainment fix.

I will also be adding audio meditations around scripture on the website that you'll be able to download and listen to.

You are invited to visit as often as you like. If you want to add material that will help us all, submit it at the site

Live your dreams!

This is my prayer for you!

May you rejoice in the Lord always May your gentleness be made known to all men the Lord is at hand.

Be anxious for nothing but in everything by prayer and supplication with thanksgiving, let your requests be made known to God... and the Peace of God which passes all understanding will guard your heart and your mind through Christ Jesus our Lord and Savior!

DARE TO BELIEVE!

About the Author

Grey McKenzie
Founder & Director
Soft Media Publishing Group

Grey is responsible for customized development of apps & security software solutions to help individuals and businesses monitor & protect the operation & use of their electronic communication devices.

Soft Media Publishing enjoys a client base of over 40,000 individuals, companies & government including members of agencies in FBI, DOS, IRS, Nasa, FDA, CAP, USDA, LOC just to name a few.